History of Risk Assessment in Toxicology

History of Toxicology and Environmental Health Series

History of Risk Assessment in Toxicology

Edited by

Sol Bobst
ToxSci Advisors, Houston, Texas, USA

Series Editor

Philip Wexler

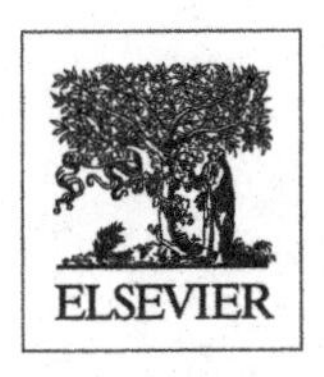

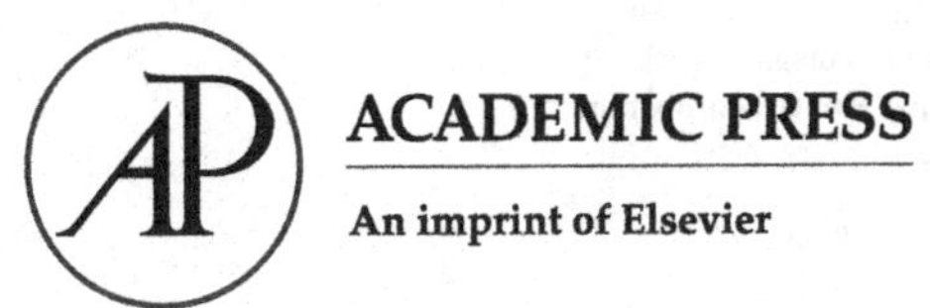

Academic Press is an imprint of Elsevier
125 London Wall, London EC2Y 5AS, United Kingdom
525 B Street, Suite 1800, San Diego, CA 92101-4495, United States
50 Hampshire Street, 5th Floor, Cambridge, MA 02139, United States
The Boulevard, Langford Lane, Kidlington, Oxford OX5 1GB, United Kingdom

Notices

Knowledge and best practice in this field are constantly changing. As new research and experience broaden our understanding, changes in research methods, professional practices, or medical treatment may become necessary.

Practitioners and researchers must always rely on their own experience and knowledge in evaluating and using any information, methods, compounds, or experiments described herein. In using such information or methods they should be mindful of their own safety and the safety of others, including parties for whom they have a professional responsibility.

To the fullest extent of the law, neither the Publisher nor the authors, contributors, or editors, assume any liability for any injury and/or damage to persons or property as a matter of products liability, negligence or otherwise, or from any use or operation of any methods, products, instructions, or ideas contained in the material herein.

British Library Cataloguing-in-Publication Data
A catalogue record for this book is available from the British Library

Library of Congress Cataloging-in-Publication Data
A catalog record for this book is available from the Library of Congress

ISBN: 978-0-12-809532-4

Publisher: Mica Haley
Acquisition Editor: Erin Hill-Parks
Editorial Project Manager: Tracy I. Tufaga
Production Project Manager: Priya Kumaraguruparan
Cover Designer: Matthew Limbert

Typeset by MPS Limited, Chennai, India

I dedicate this book to my Mother, Anne-Marie Bobst, who has always loved and supported me, even when it is challenging, and always shares love in all its forms, sweet, strong, and when necessary, . . .stinging! I love you Mom.

Your Son

Sol M. Bobst

CONTENTS

LIST OF CONTRIBUTORS

Manojit Basu
Grocery Manufacturers Association, Washington, DC, United States

Sol Bobst
ToxSci Advisors, Houston, TX, United States

Melinda Hayman
Grocery Manufacturers Association, Washington, DC, United States

Ai Kataoka
Grocery Manufacturers Association, Washington, DC, United States

Ted W. Simon
Ted Simon LLC, Winston, GA, United States

René Viñas
Grocery Manufacturers Association, Washington, DC, United States

PREFACE

"If you don't know history, then you don't know anything. You are a leaf that doesn't know it is part of a tree."—Michael Crichton

"History doesn't repeat itself, but it does rhyme."—Mark Twain

I enjoy opening a preface with these quotations about history, because they are both correct, incorrect, serious, and humorous. The History of Risk Assessment and this larger Volume Series address the compelling questions of "why things are the way they are", and "how did we get here?" I consider myself an accomplished scientist and an amateur historian. This project was humbling, because an editor and author has to decide what to include and exclude at every sentence. My hope is that future scientists interested in the history of the risk assessment discipline will take on this volume and give it added detail and narrative. We all live in a context of "doing" things. I hope that these chapters inspire the risk assessment scientist who reads them to further their own research into a historical narrative. Concepts of risk are as old as humanity. Placing a wager, or winning something based on an action, or facing grave consequences, is as old as the practice of communication. As civilizations developed, the need for decision-makers to decide how to address and protect human health has evolved with our natural and technological understanding, and capability to make decisions. The narrative of this volume starts with some of the influential events before risk assessment was practiced in earnest, and then the origins of risk assessment from the 18th century, to the emerging issues of the 21st century and the globalization and harmonization efforts of risk assessment practices. This volume has been as inclusive of relevant history as the editor and authors were able to describe in the time and character limits allowed. Any omissions noticed by the reader are encouraged to be brought to the attention of the editors. I am eternally grateful to all the chapter authors, as well as the publishing staff and their patience with me completing this project during a time of transition.

Enjoy the "Story"

Sol Bobst, PhD DABT

May 24, 2017

SERIES INTRODUCTION

In the realm of communicating any science, history, though critical to its progress, is typically a neglected backwater. This is unfortunate, as it can easily be the most fascinating, revealing, and accessible aspect of a subject which might otherwise hold appeal for only a highly specialized technical audience. Toxicology, the science concerned with the potentially hazardous effects of chemical, biological, and certain physical agents, has yet to be the subject of a full-scale historical treatment. Overlapping with many other sciences, it both draws from and contributes to them. Chemistry, biology, and pharmacology all intersect with toxicology. While there have been chapters devoted to history in toxicology textbooks, and journal articles have filled in bits and pieces of the historical record, this new monographic series aims to further remedy the gap by offering an extensive and systematic look at the subject from antiquity to the present.

Since ancient times, men and women have sought security of all kinds. This includes identifying and making use of beneficial substances while avoiding the harmful ones, or mitigating harm already caused. Thus, food and other natural products, independently or in combination, which promoted well-being or were found to have drug-like properties and effected cures, were readily consumed, applied, or otherwise self-administered or made available to friends and family. On the other hand, agents found to cause injury or damage—what we might call *poisons* today—were personally avoided although sometimes employed to wreak havoc upon one's enemies.

While natural substances are still of toxicological concern, synthetic and industrial chemicals now predominate as the emphasis of research. Through the years, the instinctive human need to seek safety and avoid hazard has served as an unchanging foundation for toxicology, and will be explored from many angles in this series. Although largely examining the scientific underpinnings of the field, chapters will also delve into the fascinating history of toxicology and poisons in mythology, arts, society, and culture more broadly. It is a subject that has captured our collective consciousness.

The series is intentionally broad, thus the title *History of Toxicology and Environmental Health*. Clinical and research toxicology, environmental and occupational health, risk assessment, and epidemiology, to name but a few examples, are all fair game subjects for inclusion. Volumes 1 and 2 focus on toxicology in antiquity, taken roughly to be the period up to the fall of the Roman empire and stopping short of the Middle Ages, with which period future volumes will continue. These opening volumes will explore toxicology from the perspective of some of the great civilizations of the past, including Egypt, Greece, Rome, Mesoamerica, and China. Particular substances, such as harmful botanicals, lead, cosmetics, kohl, and hallucinogens, serve as the focus of other chapters. The role of certain individuals as either victims or practitioners of toxicity (e.g., Cleopatra, Mithridates, Alexander the Great, Socrates, and Shen Nung) serves as another thrust of these volumes.

History proves that no science is static. As Nikola Tesla said, "The history of science shows that theories are perishable. With every new truth that is revealed we get a better understanding of Nature and our conceptions and views are modified."

Great research derives from great researchers who do not, and cannot, operate in a vacuum, but rely on the findings of their scientific forebears. To quote Sir Isaac Newton, "If I have seen further it is by standing on the shoulders of giants."

Welcome to this toxicological journey through time. You will surely see further and deeper and more insightfully by wafting through the waters of toxicology's history.

Phil Wexler

CHAPTER 1

Prehistory of Risk Assessment: Origins of Human Tragedies and Concepts of Risk

Sol Bobst
ToxSci Advisors, Houston, TX, United States

1.1 INTRODUCTION

In modern human civilization, the devastation caused by human disease, war, and natural disasters is well documented. Some discussion of these topics is warranted in an introduction to the history of risk assessment, to set the stage for defining and understanding what risk was. The following table below shows some of the devastating illnesses, the times they were noted, and the death toll they created.

Disease	Timeline	Death Toll
Tuberculosis	Prerecorded time	Unknown > Millions
Influenza	4000 BC–Present	Unknown > Millions
Malaria	3000 BC–Present	Unknown > Million
Bubonic plague	500/1300 AD	>25 million people
Measles	800 AD –Present	> Hundreds of thousands
Typhus	1400–1500 AD	> Hundreds of thousands
Chicken pox	1500 AD	Unknown > Millions
Yellow fever	1500 to present	> Hundreds of thousands
Small pox	1500 BC–20th century	> 7 million people (Roman Epidemic)

These tragedies and experiences helped to develop the idea of adverse outcomes and the need for responding to public health needs. While medicine would take several centuries to modernize to address sanitation in health, these human experiences are noteworthy in the development of ideas of risk.

History of Risk Assessment in Toxicology. DOI: http://dx.doi.org/10.1016/B978-0-12-809532-4.00001-1

1.2 THE MATHEMATICAL DEVELOPMENT OF RISK CONCEPTS

Before there was a concept of risk, there were concepts of the mathematical ideas around chance. Some of the first to document principles of probability include Girolamo Cardano (1500–71) who wrote a book titled *Liber de Ludo Aleae* (*Books on Game of Chance*). John Graunt published a compilation on the birth and death records in London from 1604 to 1661 titled *The Natural and Political Observations made upon the Bills of Mortality*. Thus, this was a historical example of how often an unwanted outcome in death or birth may happen as a rate of occurrence within a larger population, or show any trends or changes over a period of time.

1.3 PERCIVALL POTT AND CHIMNEY SWEEPERS

An important milestone in any risk assessment history timeline would have to include Percivall Pott's study of chimney sweepers and the incidence of Soot wart (skin cancer on the scrotum). It is known as the first documented case of occupationally related cancer. This work was published in 1775. By 1778, the British Parliament passed an act where children engaged in chimney sweep work should be required to take a bath at least once a week, in order to remove soot from their body, which Percivall had suggested was an associated or causative agent in the development of the warts, and if continuingly irritated, the development of scrotal cancer. The historical importance of Pott's work was directly helpful in responding the Spinner's Mule Cancers a little over 100 years later in 1890, where the spinner would use mineral oil in the occupation, and the soot also resulted in scrotal cancer. This helped continue a trend of associated exposure with effect, and the management of the risk by controlling the occupational environment, or by changing hygiene practices.

1.4 INDUSTRIAL SMOG AND REGULATORY RESPONSES

The distribution of electric power that came from coal-fired power for steam, and then eletrical power plants in the early-to-late 1800s resulted in some written descriptions of London smog in the Victorian era, like that of Flora Tristan in the *London Journal*, who wrote in 1839: "Over every English town there hangs a pall compounded of the Ocean vapours that perpetually shroud the British Isles, and the heavy noxious fumes of the Cyclops' cave". Another famous documentation of industrial pollution is Monet's painting of London looking at Parliament in 1899 that appeared to give the impression of smog. The Industrial Revolution thus caused smog conditions around many population centers globally. One well known tragedy of this smog without regulation was the great "Smog of London" which occurred from December 5–9, in 1952. This was a result of the heavy coal emissions combined with a period of cold weather, anticyclone, and windless conditions resulting in respiratory ailments that caused 4000–12,000 deaths, and over 100,000 became sick or were hospitalized with respiratory illnesses. The response was the passing of the Clean Air Act in 1956 and 1958, which provided financial incentives for individual homes to not use coal to heat their homes; it is suggested that it took up to 10 years to observe a notable change in air quality in the city of London. Air pollution continues to be a problem for major metropolitan areas, such as Beijing and other cities in China, with large industrial complexes as well as automotive traffic filling the air with particulates and other forms of soot. Air quality and regulation continues to be an challenge for policy makers and industrial/community stakeholders to manage to improve health and quality of life.

1.5 THE NARRATIVE OF THE HISTORY OF TOXICOLOGICAL RISK ASSESSMENT

This book is admittedly narrow in scope, but this is also due to the fact that toxicological risk assessment is a niche practice by definition. However, the practice of risk assessment spans several industries, including food, industrial chemicals, consumer products, and pharmaceutical development. From a historical perspective, this book addresses the narrative of how legislation and risk assessment practices have developed over time. Risk assessment involves both the traditional scientific methods and development of data, and it also has a subjective element of human perception that influences how decisions are made. The book and the authors have explained the narrative of risk assessment by showing these case study examples. The narrative of this short book will illustrate to the reader how current regulations around risk assessment in the US EPA and FDA have developed, and this leads to the current topics of the emerging issues and current debates that are ongoing today, about how we as a scientific community practice risk assessment.

FURTHER READING

https://en.wikipedia.org/wiki/List_of_natural_disasters_by_death_toll.

Bernstein, P.L., 1996. Against the Gods: The Remarkable Story of Risk. Wiley, New York.

https://en.wikipedia.org/wiki/Chimney_sweeps%27_carcinoma.

http://www.mytimemachine.co.uk/?p=62.

http://www.metoffice.gov.uk/learning/learn-about-the-weather/weather-phenomena/case-studies/great-smog.

https://en.wikipedia.org/wiki/Pollution_in_China.

CHAPTER 2

Risk Assessment in the 20th Century Part I: Early Lessons in Food and Drug Safety

René Viñas, Melinda Hayman, Ai Kataoka and Manojit Basu

SECTION 2.1

Food Additives and Contaminants

René Viñas
Grocery Manufacturers Association, Washington, DC, United States

2.1.1 INTRODUCTION

Conducting risk evaluations for food is unique, primarily because of the complexity of food itself as well as the role that food plays as a central focus in many cultures. An individual may eat more than 1 kg of food a day, which would be equivalent to approximately 30 tons of food and about 5330 kg of direct food additives over a lifetime (82 years) (Lane, 2016). Considering the large intake of food by an individual, the top priority of regulatory agencies and food manufacturers is to ensure that the appropriate safety measures are taken, whether it is for food additives, genetically modified organisms (GMOs), or the prevention of bacterial contamination. The aim of this chapter is to provide the reader with a brief overview of how risk assessment is applied to food safety.

2.1.2 FOOD ADDITIVES

Food additives serve a number of purposes such as food preservation, maintaining freshness, preventing bacterial contamination, enhancing taste, and improving nutritional value, amongst many others (FDA). According to Section 201(s) of the Federal Food, Drug, and Cosmetic Act (FFDCA), a food additive is defined as "any substance the intended use of which results or may reasonably be expected to result,

History of Risk Assessment in Toxicology. DOI: http://dx.doi.org/10.1016/B978-0-12-809532-4.00002-3

directly or indirectly, in its becoming a component or otherwise affecting the characteristics of any food". Substances included in the definition include the intended use in producing, manufacturing, packaging, processing, transporting, and/or food storage (21CFR170.3).

Food additives are subject to authorization by the U.S. FDA, with authorization only being granted provided that the additive in question is safe under the principle of "reasonable certainty of no harm" (FDA (a)). Establishing an additive as safe means that the intended use of a substance is not harmful as determined by competent scientists (21CFR170.3). According to the Code of Federal Regulations Title 21, in order to determine safety the following factors must be considered:

1. The probable consumption of the substance and of any substance formed in or on food because of its use.
2. The cumulative effect of the substance in the diet, taking into account any chemically or pharmacologically related substance or substances in such diet.
3. Safety factors which, in the opinion of experts qualified by scientific training and experience to evaluate the safety of food and food ingredients, are generally recognized as appropriate.

The U.S. FDA provides the *Toxicological Principles for the Safety Assessment of Direct Food Additives and Color Additives Used in Food*, commonly known as the "Redbook", as a guide for industry and the public concerning procedures and methodologies for conducting safety assessments (FDA, 1982). The Redbook provides guidance on the U.S. FDA's expectations in regards to premarket approval such as: identifying the appropriate toxicological studies; identifying potential human health effects from exposure to ingredients; as well as designing, performing, and reporting safety assessment conclusions from toxicological studies. At the time of this writing, the U.S. FDA is in the process of revising and updating the Redbook due to advances in toxicological methodologies.

The primary purpose of a risk assessment for a food additive is to derive an acceptable daily intake (ADI). Based on animal studies, an ADI is calculated from the dose level after the chronic ingestion of the additive that was shown to cause a no adverse effect level (NOAEL), and by the application of the appropriate safety factors (FDA, 1982). Safety factors typically applied include species differences and individual differences (i.e., genetic variability). Usually, a safety factor of 100 is applied as a default (Tralau et al., 2015). The food additive in question is usually considered safe for its intended use as long as the estimated daily intake (EDI) is less than the ADI, whereby the EDI takes into account: (1) the concentration of an additive in food, and (2) the consumers' food intake that will or might contain the substance (FDA, 1982).

2.1.3 FOOD CONTAMINANTS

Contaminants in food are by definition unwanted substances. Food contaminants can be naturally occurring, such as mycotoxins, while still others can be process-form related such as acrylamide. Food contaminants can also be introduced at any point of the supply chain, such as during the manufacturing, preparation, and packaging, or during transport. In any case, to assess an adverse effect from a contaminant one has to determine the tolerable daily intake (TDI), which is the estimated quantity of a chemical substance that can be ingested daily over a lifetime without causing a significant risk to human health (EFSA, 2015). Similarly to the ADI, the TDI is calculated from NOAELs or benchmark dose (BMD) values derived from animal studies and taking into consideration the appropriate safety factors (Tralau et al., 2015). To estimate exposure, databases of food intake such as the National Health and Nutrition Examination Survey (NHANES) are typically used in order to estimate consumption patterns of the respective food of concern (NHANES). If there is a deficiency in chemical-specific toxicity data, the threshold of toxicological concern (TTC) can be applied. The TTC is based on structural and functional categorizations of chemicals derived from years of animal studies and a variety of chemicals with the intent of informing risk managers whether exposure levels are low enough to make further gathering of additional data unnecessary, or to prioritize substances for further testing (Canady et al., 2013; EFSA, 2016; Kroes et al., 2005).

2.1.4 CHALLENGES

Several challenges exist when it comes to conducting a risk assessment for food safety. One example is the development and implementation of methodologies for evaluating mixture toxicity and cumulative exposure to structurally relate substances, as well as for substances that share a common mechanism of action (Tralau et al., 2015).

Other challenges include access to limited food consumption and occurrence data to conduct a robust exposure assessment for additives and contaminants; there is also the need for further refinement of strategies for the assessment of potential epigenetic effects, endocrine disruptors, and the use of novel material such as nanoparticles.

REFERENCES

21CFR170.3. Code of Federal Regulations Title 21, Volume 3. Available at: <https://www.accessdata.fda.gov/scripts/cdrh/cfdocs/cfcfr/CFRSearch.cfm?fr=170.3&SearchTerm=additive>.

Canady, R., Lane, R., Paoli, G., Wilson, M., Bialk, H., Hermansky, S., et al., 2013. Determining the applicability of threshold of toxicological concern approaches to substances found in foods. Crit. Rev. Food Sci. Nutr. 53, 1239–1249.

EFSA. 2015. EFSA explains the safety of Bisphenol A. Available at: <https://www.efsa.europa.eu/en/topics/factsheets/factsheetbpa150121>.

EFSA. 2016. Review of the Threshold of Toxicological Concern (TTC) approach and development of new TTC decision tree. European food Safety Authority and World Health Organization. Question number: EFSA-Q-2016-00080. (1–42).

FDA (a). Federal Food, Drug, and Cosmetic Act. Available at: <http://www.fda.gov/RegulatoryInformation/Legislation/FederalFoodDrugandCosmeticActFDCAct/default.htm>.

FDA, 1982. Toxicological Principles for the Safety Assessment of Direct Food Additives and Color Additives used in Food. U.S. Food and Drug Administration, Bureau of Foods, Washington, DC. Available at: http://www.fda.gov/Food/GuidanceRegulation/GuidanceDocumentsRegulatoryInformation/IngredientsAdditivesGRASPackaging/ucm2006826.htm.

Kroes, R., Kleiner, J., Renwick, A., 2005. The threshold of toxicological concern concept in risk assessment. Toxicol. Sci. 86 (2), 226–230. Available from: http://dx.doi.org/10.1093/toxsci/kfi169.

Lane, R., 2016. Food toxicology lecture. Advanced comprehensive toxicology course. American College of Toxicology.

NHANES. National Health and Nutrition Examination Survey. Available at: <https://www.cdc.gov/nchs/nhanes/>.

Tralau, T., Oelgeschläger, M., Gürtler, R., Heinemeyer, G., Herzler, M., Höfer, T., et al., 2015. Regulatory toxicology in the twenty-first century: challenges, perspectives and possible solutions. Arch. Toxicol. 89, 823–850. Available from: http://dx.doi.org/10.1007/s00204-015-1510-0.

SECTION 2.2
Microbial Risk Assessment

Melinda Hayman and Ai Kataoka
Grocery Manufacturers Association, Washington, DC, United States

Foodborne disease caused by pathogenic microorganisms is a global concern. Due to the underlying complexity associated with the modern food supply system, it is crucial for risk managers to take a scientifically sound and systematic approach to evaluate the risks associated with food. Emerging microbial food safety hazards constantly arise due to new agricultural practices, changing food processing technologies, the global nature and complexity of the food supply system, and new consumer trends. In addition, microbes continually evolve, and there is variability in the virulence and pathogenicity within a genus or a species. Therefore, control strategies and measures need to be re-reviewed and updated as new food safety issues emerge. Risk assessment has been utilized in the area of food microbiology as a tool to ensure food safety and public health. This approach allows the risk manager to make appropriate decisions and establish effective control measures. This section discusses the history and applications of risk assessment in the field of food microbiology.

The food microbiology community adopted risk assessment in late 1990s, after observing success in the field of food chemistry in the 1980s. It rapidly established credibility and utility in the field of food microbiology, largely due to a relationship with international policy and trade. In 1995, the agreement on the Application of Sanitary and Phytosanitary Measures (known as the SPS Agreement) was implemented with the World Trade Organization (WTO) to ensure food safety, as well as plant and animal health, among member countries. The agreement states that any measurements utilized to achieve the objectives of the agreement should be based on decisions derived from a risk assessment (WTO). Subsequently, there have been efforts to establish internationally harmonized guidance to conduct risk assessments within the Food and Agriculture Organization of the United Nations (FAO) together with the World Health Organization (WHO).

The Codex Alimentarius Commission (Codex) developed their guidance document "Principles and Guidelines for the Conduct of Microbiological Risk Assessment" in 1999 (Codex, 1999), which has been considered to be the gold standard among the risk assessment community. The FAO/WHO and Codex lead developing guidance documents related to risk analysis and performing risk assessments for certain hazards and food commodities, such as "Risk assessment of *Listeria monocytogenes* in ready-to-eat foods" (FAO/WHO, 2004), and "Risk assessment of *Vibrio parahaemolyticus* in seafood" (FAO/WHO, 2011). The Codex Committee on Food Hygiene (CCFH) has developed guidelines related to microbial risk assessments and a risk analysis framework. Additionally, advances in computing capability have further contributed to the advancement of risk assessment through the ability to analyze and comprehend complex and dynamic data associated with microorganisms (i.e., predictive mathematical models). Although comprehensive risk assessment can be used by any organization, institution, or companies other than international organizations or government bodies, the resources and discipline necessary to carry out the process appropriately could be hurdles for smaller scale organizations.

As mentioned above, the Codex guideline is the gold standard among international food safety communities, and provides definitions of key words and explains approaches to performing risk assessments (Codex, 1999). According to the document, a risk assessment is defined as:

> *a scientifically based process consisting of the following steps: (i) hazard identification, (ii) hazard characterization, (iii) exposure assessment, and (iv) risk characterization.*

Each step can be briefly described as follows (Codex, 1999):

- Hazard identification is a step to identify pathogenic microbial agents in food,
- Hazard characterization is to describe the adverse health effect qualitatively or quantitatively caused by the pathogenic microbial agents including dose response,
- Exposure assessment is to evaluate outcomes of human exposure to the pathogenic microbial agents, and
- Risk characterization is to incorporate all of above to conclude a risk estimate.

Two types of risk assessments were defined as follows (Codex, 1999):

- Quantitative Risk Assessment – A Risk Assessment that provides numerical expressions of risk and an indication of the attendant uncertainties (stated in the 1995 Expert Consultation definition on Risk Analysis).
- Qualitative Risk Assessment – A Risk Assessment based on data which, while forming an inadequate basis for numerical risk estimations, nonetheless, when conditioned by prior expert knowledge and identification of attendant uncertainties permits risk ranking or separation into descriptive categories of risk.

Quantitative risk assessments in food microbiology present numerical outcomes on the likelihood of adverse health consequences from hazards of concern derived from data using mathematical models to incorporate illness data, dose response, an organism's growth characteristics, and food consumption information. The quantitative risk assessment can be further divided into two categories: probabilistic and deterministic risk assessments. The probabilistic approach considers all possible scenarios, likelihoods, and associated impacts of a hazard, whereas the deterministic approach rather takes single-point estimates, with a value of risk that is most representative, and typically at a worst case scenario. Where possible, the probabilistic approach is preferred. The output of qualitative risk assessment may be demonstrated with comparative terminology (i.e., high, medium, or low risk). Risk assessors will chose a type of risk assessment to be developed based on a hazard of concerns, a food type, and data and resources available.

Risk assessment for food microbiology hazards differs from that for chemical hazards; a key difference is due to the fact that microbial hazards are living organisms and grow in a food matrix and/or a host. Growth, survival, and death of microorganisms are affected by a type of organism (i.e., genus/species and even strain), as well as the intrinsic and extrinsic factors associated with the food or environment. Furthermore, infected individuals may become a source of further contamination and infection. Susceptibility to certain pathogenic organisms differs in the population. Individuals with a weakened immune system (i.e., young children, the elderly, and immuno-compromised individuals) are known to develop more severe adverse health consequences upon exposure to certain microbial pathogens. An infectious

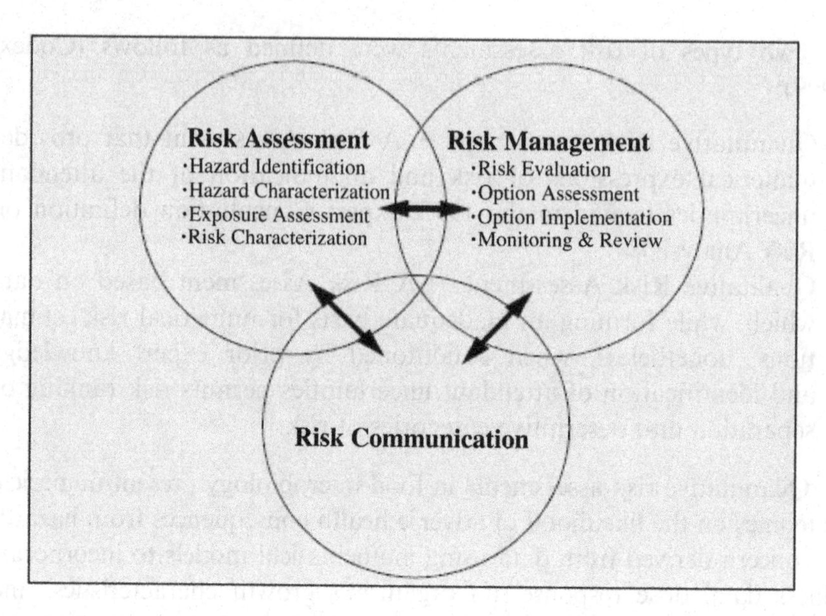

Figure 2.2.1 Risk analysis framework for food microbiology. Adapted from FAO/WHO. 1997. Risk Management and Food Safety. Report of a Joint FAO/WHO Consultation. Rome, Italy, 27–31 January 1997. FAO, Rome.

dose may differ depending on the immune status of the host. Therefore, dose response or exposure assessment becomes much more challenging compared to chemical risk assessments. Accordingly, the outcomes of microbial risk assessment may be more complex and not as clear as the numerical output seen in chemical assessments (i.e., a minimum dose of a certain food additive).

Risk analysis, which consists of risk assessment, risk management, and risk communication (Fig. 2.2.1), has been utilized, especially for international organizations and government bodies, to develop guidelines and standards to enhance food safety and public health. Risk managers utilize outcomes from risk assessment to develop control measures (i.e., standards, guidelines, or regulations) and to allocate resources effectively. As mentioned above, microbial risk assessment is complex, and it has been recognized that exploiting an outcome to develop such control measures is often not straightforward. The FAO/WHO and Codex have been working to develop guidelines regarding risk management frameworks based on microbial risk assessment outputs. In 2007, Codex published the guidance document (Codex, 2007) and a diagram is presented to demonstrate an overview of the concept (Fig. 2.2.2). This approach will enhance applications of risk assessment outcomes effectively.

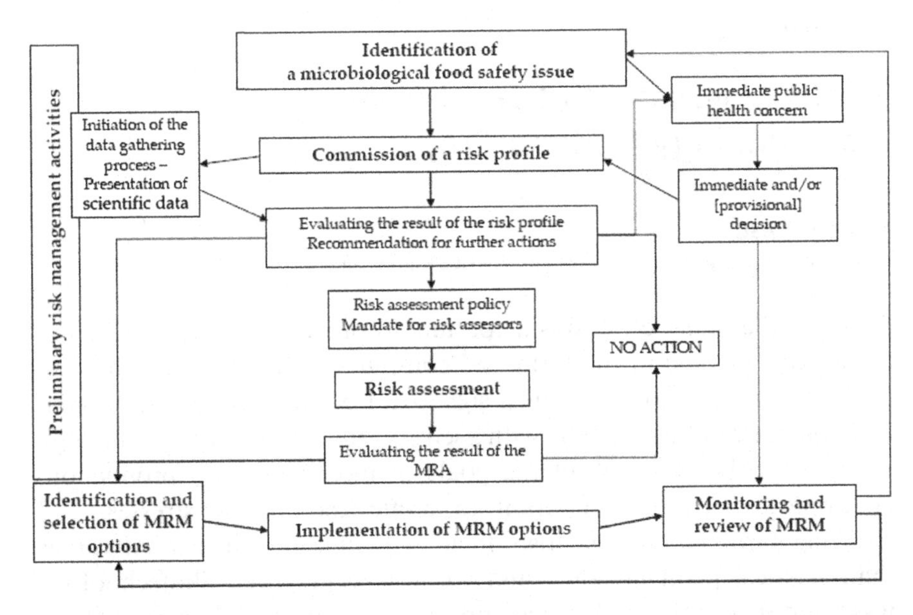

Figure 2.2.2 Diagrammatic overview of the microbial risk management framework (from the Draft Codex Principle and Guidelines for the Conduct of Microbiological Risk Management). Adapted from FAO/WHO, 2006. The use of microbiological risk assessment outputs to develop practical risk management strategies: metrics to improve food safety. Report of a Joint FAO/WHO Expert Meeting. FAO. Rome.

REFERENCES

Codex Alimentarius Commission, 1999. Principles and guidelines for the conduct of microbiological risk assessment. CAC/GL 30-1999. Adopted 1999. Amendments 2012, 2014.

Codex Alimentarius Commission, 2007. Principles and guidelines for the conduct of microbiological risk management (MRM) Annex II: Guidance on Microbiological Risk Management Metrics.

FAO/WHO, 1997. Risk management and food safety. Report of a Joint FAO/WHO Consultation. Rome, Italy, 27–31 January 1997. FAO, Rome.

FAO/WHO, 2004. Risk assessment of *Listeria monocytogenes* in ready-to-eat foods. Available at: <ftp://ftp.fao.org/docrep/fao/010/y5394e/y5394e.pdf> (accessed 25.10.16).

FAO/WHO, 2006. The use of microbiological risk assessment outputs to develop practical risk management strategies: metrics to improve food safety. Report of a Joint FAO/WHO Expert Meeting. FAO. Rome.

FAO/WHO, 2011. Risk assessment of *Vibrio parahaemolyticus* in seafood. Available at: <http://apps.who.int/iris/bitstream/10665/44566/1/9789241548175_eng.pdf?ua = 1> (accessed 25.10.16).

World Trade Organization. Sanitary and phytosanitary measures: text of the agreement. The WTO Agreement on the Application of Sanitary and Phytosanitary Measures (SPS Agreement). Available at: <https://www.wto.org/english/tratop_e/sps_e/spsagr_e.htm> (accessed 11.10.16).

SECTION 2.3

Safety Assessment of Food from Biotechnology-Derived Crops

Manojit Basu
Grocery Manufacturers Association, Washington, DC, United States

Ensuring the safety of food is a continuous process, and it starts before a seed gets planted in the farm and continues till the food reaches the plate. Agriculture holds the most significant position in our food chain, and commercial farming has witnessed the advent of a new technology since the early 1990s. With the goals of increasing crop production, developing crops more tolerant to biotic and abiotic stresses, and reducing farm inputs, scientists focused their research in areas other than classical plant breeding and agronomic practices. Biotechnology was identified as the tool to accomplish the goals of feeding an increasing population and meeting the demands of commercial agriculture. The first biotechnology-derived crop reached the market in 1994, when the delayed ripening tomato (Flavr Savr) was introduced (Krieger et al., 2008).

The safety of food from biotechnology-derived crops is ensured through robust and science based assessment criteria which use the concept of "substantial equivalence" (Society of Toxicology, 2003). This concept relies on comparing the new plant variety to its traditional counterpart in terms of safety and nutrition. This section will focus on product characterization conducted to ensure the safety of biotechnology-derived crops.

Product characterization for ensuring safety is a two-step process which lasts almost the length of the product development life-cycle. For biotechnology-derived crops, the time to market can be close to a decade or more, based on the crop. The first step in the process begins early during the discovery stage, when researchers are involved in identifying the gene of interest that they want to introduce into a plant. During discovery stage, the focus is on ensuring that the gene of interest does not code for a protein which is a known allergen, toxin, or protein demonstrating an adverse biological effect. Once the safety of the transgene is established and the transgene is inserted in to a new plant, several years of field testing are carried out to ensure that the gene of interest is efficacious, and that the plant is agronomically and physiologically similar to its nontransformed counterpart.

The second step of the safety assessment is most critical and relies heavily on molecular characterization, proteolytic stability, and animal feeding studies. Molecular characterization is carried out to identify the location of the transgene insertion in the host genome, the number of copies of the transgene inserted, and to obtain the nucleotide sequence of the transgene and the flanks at both ends as it got inserted in the plant. The sequence data is used to conduct a suite of bioinformatics analyses which include determining the structural similarity, sequence homology, and serological identity of the transgene as it is inserted in a plant with known allergens, toxins, and adverse proteins. Additionally, proteolytic stability studies are conducted to determine the resistance of the transgene encoded protein from breaking down when exposed to gastric acids, which is important to determine the allergenic potential of the protein under investigation. Last but not least, animal feeding studies are conducted using the protein extracted from the transgenic plant to evaluate the toxicity and carcinogenicity of the protein across several animal models. These feeding studies are short- and long-duration studies similar to toxicological studies used to ensure the safety of food additives. Finally, to ensure that a biotechnology-derived crop remains safe, the bioinformatics analyses conducted to determine similarity to known allergens, toxins, and adverse proteins need to be repeated every year and reported to the regulatory agencies as per registration requirements.

REFERENCES

Krieger, E.K., Allen, E., Gilbertson, L.A., Roberts, J.K., Hiatt, W., Sanders, R.A., 2008. The flavr savr tomato, an early example of RNAi technology. Hortic. Sci. 43 (3), 962–964.

Society of Toxicology Executive Summary, 2003. The safety of genetically modified foods produced through biotechnology. Toxicol. Sci. 71 (1), 2–8.

CHAPTER 3

History of European and Global Regulation of Risk Assessment

Sol Bobst
ToxSci Advisors, Houston, TX, United States

The introductory chapter of this book discussed the story of Percival Pott's research on scrotal cancer and chimney sweepers in Britain, which led to legislation that required chimney sweepers to receive a bath at least once a week. This 18th century risk assessment is an early example of managing risk. This chapter will include central European authority histories, as well as other global entities and the emergence of risk assessment programs around the globe. The narrative of risk assessment history is that as science and business enterprise have become global, so are the expectations of high standards in scientific and ethical integrity for risk assessment and management of chemical safety, to protect workers, the general public, consumers, and the environment. The early 21st century includes some centralization of governing authorities under the European Union.

3.1 KEY DEVELOPMENTS IN THE 1960S

The 1960s was an active time in Europe, parallel with new environmental and health regulations being developed in earnest in the United States. The post-World War II market included the development of nuclear power, which required safety studies in order to keep researchers and industrial workers safe. This also led to the development of international study groups under the World Health Organization, which has a strong presence in Europe. The sections below discuss the development of frameworks and structures that influenced the use and practice of risk assessment by regulatory bodies in Europe, and now globally.

History of Risk Assessment in Toxicology. DOI: http://dx.doi.org/10.1016/B978-0-12-809532-4.00005-9

3.2 WORLD HEALTH ORGANIZATION

The first meeting of the World Health Assembly was in 1948 in Geneva, Switzerland. It is now in its 70th year as of 2017 and has grown from 55 member states to 194 member states. The assembly is the governing forum for the World Health Organization (WHO) located in Paris, France. Part of the WHO charge, is to develop international health regulations, which includes chemicals classification and the development of the International Agency for Research on Cancer (IARC).

3.3 WHO–IARC

Several French leaders and public health figures influenced Charles De Gaulle to start a project to address the ever-growing burden of cancer. During the World Health Assembly in Geneva, Switzerland in May of 1965, the International Agency for Research on Cancer was launched. Some highlights related to the development of Risk Assessment are sourced from the epublication "IARC the first 50 years". The early years of IARC were led by epidemiologists and there was particular interest in the work of Johanness Clemensen who started the first National Cancer Registry in Denmark. Data that compared trends in the incidence of cervical cancer in Copenhagen, Denmark were compared to data from Verona, Italy. Statistical data organized and led by epidemiologists continued through the 1960s, until Richard Doll's book in 1967 titled *Prevention in Cancer: Pointers from Epidemiology*, which started to point to the associations of chemical exposure as well as chemical, physical, and biological agents. With the recognition that laboratory tests with animals were as important as epidemiological studies suggesting associations, this led to the creation in 1969 of the IARC Monograph program, which collected scientists to form working groups to assess carcinogenic hazards from occupational, environmental, and lifestyle exposures and agents. The IARC classification system has become very influential in the regulatory application of listing or classifying carcinogens. Updates to the IARC classification can have a major economic impact with market restrictions and precautionary protocols. The IARC classification is recommended and finalized by the working group, which reads available and relevant research relevant to exposure. Research efforts by various stakeholders, then, maybe targeted to influence the IARC classification or working group decision and outcome. Thus, the operation and evolution of the IARC process is an important narrative that influences the hazard classification/categorization of carcinogens, and the practice or application of risk assessment globally for it.

3.4 WHO–IPCS

The World Health Organization also administers the International Program on Chemcial Safety. The project was initiated after the 1992 meeting of the United Nations Conference on Environment and Development (UNCED), held in Rio in 1992, and subsequently "Priorities for Action Resolution" of the International Forum on Chemical Safety (IFCS) was adopted in 1994. The UNCED recommendation was reconfirmed at the 2002 World Summit on Sustainable Development, in Johannesburg. In 2005, the project produced a strategic work plan and many publications have been produced since. A further summary of this can be accessed at: http://www.who.int/ipcs/methods/harmonization/en/brochurefinal.pdf

3.5 DANGEROUS SUBSTANCE DIRECTIVE

In 1967, while the WHO was in its infancy and public awareness was rising with respect to chemical exposure and adverse health outcomes, the European Economic Community passed legislation that was adopted by member organizations for the uniform classification, packaging, and labeling of chemicals (Council Directive, 1967). Commonly referred to as the Dangerous Substance Directive, officially called the Council Directive 67/548/EE, this included classification of physical-, human-health and biological-environmental hazards. One significant update to the law occurred in 1992 which required that "risk assessments" be carried out on any new chemicals that required classification and labeling (Commission Directive, 1993; Commission Regulation, 1994). This aligned with the practice of Risk Assessment by the US EPA in the early years of its IRIS program. After receiving several updates to the law over the decades, the general legislation was replaced in 2009 as part of the new Registration, Evaluation, Authorization, of Chemicals (REACH) legislation, with the Classification, Labelling, and Packaging Law taking effect in January of 2009. The new regulation included the recently released Globally Harmonized System (GHS) of Classification and Labeling developed by the United Nations (UN).

3.6 RISK ASSESSMENT UNDER REACH

In 2003, the EU *Technical Guidance Document on Risk Assessment* provided general principles of risk assessment, and, importantly, technical details on how to perform a chemical risk assessment. The EU REACH Regulation (2006) provides the current regulatory framework for risk assessment of chemicals manufactured or imported into the EU. Specifically, REACH sets out how importers and manufacturers are to assess and document risks that arise during the manufacture and use of chemicals, as well as how to adequately control any identified risks.

The REACH (Registration, Evaluation, Authorisation and Restriction of Chemicals) Regulation (1907/2006/EC) came into force on June 1, 2007, and represents the current EU regulatory framework on risk assessment of all chemical substances manufactured or imported into the EU in quantities ≥1 tonne/year. As in all standard risk assessment processes for chemicals, REACH human health risk assessments involve both the determination of the hazard(s) posed by the chemical as well as exposure assessment (known, estimated or modeled). Annex I of REACH sets out how manufacturers and importers are to assess, and document, the risks arising from the substance(s) they manufacture or import are adequately controlled during manufacture and their own use(s) and that others further down the supply chain can adequately control the risks. Annex I states that one objective of the human health hazard assessment (which is one component of the chemical safety assessment; CSA) is "... to derive levels of exposure to the substance above which humans should not be exposed. This level of exposure is known as the Derived No-Effect Level (DNEL)." In ECHA's REACH guidance, the DNEL has been defined as "... the level of exposure above which humans should not be exposed."

3.7 OECD

The Organization for Economic Development and Cooperation came into existence on September 30, 1961. This came from the charge of the Organization for European Economic Cooperation and Development. OEECD that was created in 1948 after World War II to administer the Marshall Plan. In a council decision in 1987, member countries decided to establish or strengthen national programs to systematically investigate existing chemicals. Then through another OECD council decision in 1991, member countries agreed to investigate existing chemicals in a cooperative way, and to focus on high production volume (HPV) chemicals based on the assumption that production volume is a surrogate for data on occupational, consumer and environmental exposure (Council Acts, 1987, 1991). Each country agreed to share the burden of assessing HPV chemicals by sponsoring a proportion of the HPV chemicals in the program. By sharing work, countries and industries have benefitted from the assessments conducted by other members.

In 1998, the global chemical industry, through the International Council of Chemical Associations (ICCA) initiative, announced its intention to work with OECD by using the OECD HPV chemicals list to establish a working list of approximately 1000 substances as priorities for investigation based on presumed wide dispersive use, production in two or more global regions or similarity to another chemical meeting either of these criteria. To significantly increase the output of the program and make best use of the industry initiatives, a major refocusing was agreed by OECD member countries in 1998 with the aim of increasing transparency, efficiency and productivity and allow longer-term planning for governments and industries. Therefore, the OECD work began to focus on initial hazard assessments of HPV chemicals and no longer included extensive exposure information gathering and evaluation. Instead, detailed exposure assessments could be conducted within national (or regional) programmes and priority setting activities as post-SIDS work. During the late 1990s, member countries also began to assess groups of chemicals (chemical categories) and use (Q)SAR results, spurring the creation of OECD guidance documents as well as a computerized QSAR Toolbox. Over the next few years, comprehensive chemical assessment programmes were implemented at national and regional levels. The programme therefore needed to be revised to allow member countries and other stakeholders to save more resources and to avoid duplication. This evolution also promoted integrated approaches to testing and assessment. With this new direction, the OECD HPV Chemicals Programme evolved into the OECD Cooperative Chemicals Assessment Programme to better respond to the needs of member countries.

3.8 SELECTED COUNTRIES AND REGIONS WITH VARIOUS STATES OF RISK ASSESSMENT FRAMEWORKS

3.8.1 Canada

3.8.1.1 Health Canada and Environment Canada

The Government of Canada established a decision making framework for identifying, assessing, and managing health risks in August of 2000. Environment Canada manages toxic substances under the Canadian Environmental Protection Act, or CEPA 1999. Risk Management is regulated under the Assessment of Substances section of CEPA 1999. The Domestic Substance List (DSL) maintains the inventories of substances that are considered to pose a threat to human- or environmental health. The Canadian regulatory frameworks are well developed, with science-based approaches. The reader can find more information at the following hyperlinked websites. Health Canada Decision Making Framework: http://www.hc-sc.gc.ca/ahc-asc/pubs/hpfb-dgpsa/risk-risques_tc-tm-eng.php. Environment Canada Assessment of Substances CEPA 1999 http://www.ec.gc.ca/lcpe-cepa/default.asp?lang=En&n=EE479482-1&wsdoc=16C8586D-F376-5225-C45C-6EAC80B5E0B9.

3.9 ASIA PACIFIC

3.9.1 Australia

For industrial chemicals, the August Government manages chemical risk assessment through the Department of the Environment, as well as the Department of Health and Ageing. This is though through the National Industrial Chemicals Notification and Assessment Scheme (NICNAS), and the Australian Pesticides and Veterinary Medicines Authority (APVMA). Currently, the regulations are being updated by the Council of Australian Governments (COAG) Chemical Reforms.

3.9.2 New Zealand

Risk Assessment Frameworks are published and available under the Department of Food Safety and the New Zealand Environmental Protection Authority. The reader is encouraged to visit the site for more information (http://www.epa.govt.nz/). The New Zealand Environmental Protection Agency has its own historical classification system, including the Chemical Classification and Information Database (CCID) that maintain classifications according to Hazardous Substances and New Organisms (HSNO) regulations. Chemicals allowed in New Zealand are managed on the New Zealand Inventory of Chemicals (NZIoC).

3.9.3 India

India has numerous chemical legislations, and has also received global attention on chemical risk management due to the Bhopal Gas incident in 1984. Laws regulating chemicals include the Environment Act of 1986; Hazardous Chemical Rules Act of 2000; and Chemical Accidents Amendment of 1996. Currently, none of the governing ministries have managed databases or inventories.

3.9.4 Indonesia

In Indonesia, chemical regulations are managed by the Ministry of Environment; their focus appears to be on hazard management. The website for the department is http://www.menlh.go.id/.

3.9.5 China

There are several inventories of chemicals regulated in China, a searchable database is managed at this website: http://cciss.cirs-group.com/.

In 2011, the Chinese Government published Decree 591 Regulations on Safe Management of Hazardous Chemicals in China. It is a complex piece of legislation that includes multiple governing bodies. The legislation covers the Hazard Communication (GHS) requirement, new chemicals and dangerous goods, food safety, cosmetics, occupational health, plastics and plasticizers, and coatings. Chemicals will have to be registered in a China REACH style of legislation. Legislative authority experts are centered at the Chemical Registration Center (CRC) of the Ministry of Environmental Protection (MEP) and the State Administration of Work Safety (SAWS) of the National Registration Center for Chemicals. An English translation of the entire regulation is available at: http://www.cirs-reach.com/China_Chemical_Regulation/Regulations_on_Safe_Management_of_Hazardous_Chemicals_2011_English_Translation.html.

3.9.6 Philippines

The Phillippines has an Inventory of Chemicals and Chemical Substances (PICCS), which is administered by the Environmental Management Bureau.

3.9.7 Vietnam

Vietnam has been developing and updating chemical regulation laws over the past few years. In 2011, Decree No. 26/2011/ND-CP was passed that includes inventory lists and chemicals that are limited in production and trade conditions. The lists also include chemicals subject to declaration and toxic chemicals which require control slips for purchase. Decree No. 108/2008/ND-CP contains a list of banned chemicals. The government website for chemical management is under the Ministry of Industry and Trade, located here: http://www.moit.gov.vn/.

3.9.8 Japan

In Japan, chemical management and risk assessment in Japan is managed by the National Institute of Technology and Evaluation, administered under the title of Chemical Risk Information Platform, it can be accessed at this site: http://www.safe.nite.go.jp/english/db.html.

3.9.9 Korea

The Korean Ministry of Environment has established a registration, evaluation program of chemical substances very similar to the European REACH regulations. It is so similar, that it is called K-REACH (For Korea-REACH). The regulations apply to any company that will manufacture or import any chemical subject to registration at one tonne or greater on an annual basis. The registration process will include hazard evaluation and risk assessment of the chemical within one to two years of registration. For more information visit the link provided here: http://eng.me.go.kr/eng/web/index.do?menuId=167.

3.9.10 Latin American Countries

The risk assessment process is not well developed in Latin America Countries. Although the risk of exposure to different chemicals categories is mentioned in the legislation of most of the countries there is no directive that clearly indicate how to proceed with the risk assessment process. The sections below list what is currently known about legislation in Latin American Countries that incorporate the practice and application of toxicological risk assessment.

3.9.11 Brazil

The federal government of Brazil instituted in 2007 an inter-ministerial task force coordinated by the Ministry of Industrial Development and external Commerce to implement the Global Harmonizes System in Brazil. The first version of the technical document that establish the criteria for the Classification System of Danger Products was published in September 2009 by the Brazilian Association of Technical Regulation (Technical regulation 14725-2 ABNT—Associação Brasileira de Normas Técnicas). This rule applies to all pure chemicals and mixtures and aims to provide information about the safety of chemicals to human and environmental health, to indicate the procedures for labeling of chemical products, and also how to organize the safety data sheets.

3.9.12 Uruguay

Also in 2009, Uruguay incorporated the risk assessment concept to the Act 307/009 (modified by Act 346/2011) indicating the minimal requirements for the worker health protection and safety consider occupational chemical exposure risk. The Act indicates that both hazard and exposure must be taken into account in the risk assessment process. In 2011, this regulation was amended indicating that all companies included in the original decree will have six months to develop a plan for GHS implementation.

3.9.13 Mexico

In 2011, Mexico published the NMX-R-019 NMX-R-019-SCFI-2011 that sets out the criteria for classifying chemicals according to their physical-, health-, and environmental hazards (http://trabajoseguro.stps.gob.mx/trabajoseguro/boletines%20anteriores/2011/bol039/vinculos/NMX-R-019-SCFI-2011.pdf). It also provides the elements of a uniform hazard communication system for chemical products, labeling requirements, and safety data sheets. In accordance with the third edition of the Global Harmonized System of United Nations, these rules do not apply to pharmaceutical products, food additives, cosmetics, pesticide residues in food, and danger residues (http://www.unece.org/fileadmin/DAM/trans/danger/publi/ghs/ghs_rev03/Spanish/00-intro-sp.pdf; http://www.cec.org/lawdatabase/mx11.cfm?varlan=english#4). The application of this rule by the industry is not mandatory, meaning GHS can be used on a voluntary basis and is not enforced.

In Mexico, chemical substances and products are legislated by six different regulatory agencies making the legal regime governing chemical substances a complicated and often confusing subject matter. Due to the number of laws and agencies that regulate chemical substances, an Inter-Secretarial Commission for the Control of the Processing and Use of Pesticides, Fertilizers and Toxic Substances (Comisión Intersecretarial para el Control del Proceso y Uso de Plaguicidas, Fertilizantes y Sustancias Tóxicas (CICLOPLAFEST)) was created in 1987.

REFERENCES

Commission Directive 93/67/EEC of 20 July 1993. Laying down the principles for assessment of risks to man and the environment of substances notified in accordance with Council Directive 67/548/EEC. Off. J. L 227, 08/09/1993, pp. 0009–0018.

Commission Regulation (EC) No 1488/94 of 28 June 1994. Laying down the principles for the assessment of risks to man and the environment of existing substances in accordance with Council Regulation (EEC) No 793/93 (Text with EEA relevance). Off. J. L 161, 29/06/1994, pp. 0003–0011.

Council Acts, 1987, 1991. Decision-Recommendation of the Council on the Systematic Investigation of Existing Chemicals. OECD Chemical Acts: Web Reference: http://acts.oecd.org/Instruments/ShowInstrumentView.aspx?InstrumentID=56&InstrumentPID=53&Lang = en&Book=False.

Council Directive 67/548/EEC of 27 June 1967. On the approximation of laws, regulations and administrative provisions relating to the classification, packaging and labelling of dangerous substances. Off. J. L 196, 16.8.1967, pp. 1–98.

Regulation (EC) No 1907/2006 of the European Parliament and of the Council of 18 December 2006. Concerning the Registration, Evaluation, Authorisation and Restriction of Chemicals (REACH), establishing a European Chemicals Agency, amending Directive 1999/45/EC and repealing Council Regulation (EEC) No 793/93 and Commission Regulation (EC) No 1488/94 as well as Council Directive 76/769/EEC and Commission Directives 91/155/EEC, 93/67/EEC, 93/105/EC and 2000/21/EC. Off. J. L 396, 30.12.2006, pp. 1–849.

FURTHER READING

European Agency for Safety and Health at Work. <https://osha.europa.eu/en/legislation>. (accessed 2014).

European Chemicals Agency (ECHA) Guidance for Downstream Users, December 2013. <http://echa.europa.eu/> (accessed .02.14).

European Chemicals Agency (ECHA) Guidance on Information Requirements and Chemicals Safety Assessment. Chapter R.8: Characterisation of Dose [Concentration]-Response for Human Health, November 2012. <http://echa.europa.eu/> (accessed 01.14).

European Chemicals Agency (ECHA) Guidance on Information Requirements and Chemicals Safety Assessment Part A: Introduction to the Guidance Document, December 2011. <http://echa.europa.eu/> (accessed 01.14).

CHAPTER 4

The History of Risk Assessment Within OSHA and ACGIH: Asbestos Case Study

Sol Bobst
ToxSci Advisors, Houston, TX, United States

Related to risk assessment is the evaluation and control of the work environment. Industrial hygiene, as a practice to monitor and control work environments, thus deserves some attention in a historical consideration for the evolution of risk assessment. It is important to note that the formation of a professional organization predated the formation of a governmental body by several decades. This is a testament to the dedication and honorable work of private and civil servants that self-organized in order to produce guidance and protocols in order to protect public health.

This organization was first called the independent National Conference of Governmental Industrial Hygienists (NCGIH) convened on June 27, 1938, in Washington, DC. Representatives to the conference included 76 members, representing 24 states, three cities, one university, the US Public Health Service, the US Bureau of Mines, and the Tennessee Valley Authority. This meeting was the culmination of concerted efforts by John J. Bloomfield and Royd S. Sayers. In 1946, the organization changed its name to the American Conference of Governmental Industrial Hygienists (ACGIH). The Threshold Limit Values for Chemical Substances (TLV-CS) Committee was established in 1941. This group was charged with investigating, recommending, and annually reviewing exposure limits for chemical substances. It became a standing committee in 1944. Two years later, the organization adopted its first list of 148 exposure limits, then referred to as Maximum Allowable Concentrations. The term "Threshold Limit Values (TLVs)" was introduced in 1956.

History of Risk Assessment in Toxicology. DOI: http://dx.doi.org/10.1016/B978-0-12-809532-4.00004-7

4.1 THE BIRTH OF THE OCCUPATIONAL HEALTH AND SAFETY ADMINISTRATION AND THE NATIONAL INSTITUTE OF OCCUPATIONAL SAFETY AND HEALTH

The Occupational Health and Safety Administration (OSHA) was formed in 1970 as part of the Federal Government reorganization charges that came out of the Nixon Administration. At this time, the creation of OSHA included the adoption of most (if not all) of the current TLVs published by the ACGIH as part of 29 CFR 1910.1000. At the same time, in 1970 the creation of the National Institute of Occupational Safety and Health (NIOSH), a branch now administered by the Center of Disease Control (CDC), was formed. This organization published some landmark documents like the first Asbestos Guidance Document in 1971. The guidance was developed by a 13-member review committee with the engagement of three consultants. The structure of the document included the overall recommendation for an asbestos standard. This was supported by the description of the biological effects of exposure, as well as epidemiological studies, and a "correlation of biological exposure and effect." The work also included compatibility with emissions standards at the time, and the sampling methods for industrial hygienists to take for monitoring environments for asbestos.

This organization also issued the first Toxic Substance List in 1971, well before any of the actions of the EPA under the safe water drinking act. By 1974, the organization had started to publish the immediately "dangerous to life and health" (IDLH) values, and by 1977 had the authority to enter into the workplace to evaluate the management of the working environment. By 1978, a pocket guide to chemical hazards was published and there was public praise for the regulatory programs in 1985, when the Office of Technical Assessment issued a statement with evidence supporting that the Occupational Health and Safety Act had helped to reduce exposures to vinyl chloride, dust, and lead. In 1986 the agency did outreach to external organizations to include interaction with the EPA, as well as other international agencies. The hundreds of peer review guidance documents produced by NIOSH led to the OSHA revision of approximately 376 substances.

4.2 REGULATORY STANDARDS UNDER OSHA, FOLLOWING THE ASBESTOS STORY

The Occupational Health and Safety Administration followed up on the NIOSH document with their implementation and enforcement of the recommendations. Table 4.1 shows the narrative of this timeline. What is interesting to note is that revisions to standards occurred with updated studies, and updated technology used in those studies changed or updated the methods. This is noteworthy in a history of the risk

Table 4.1 Major Milestones in the History of Asbestos Regulation

Month/Year	Milestone
5/71	A 12 f/cc permissible exposure limit (PEL) for asbestos was included in 36 FR 10466
12/71	OSHA issued an emergency temporary standard (ETS) which established a PEL of 5 f/cc as an 8-h time-weighted average (TWA) and a peak exposure level of 10 f/cc
6/72	OSHA promulgated a new final standard that established an 8-h TWA PEL of 5 f/cc, and a ceiling limit of 10 f/cc
10/75	OSHA published a notice of proposed rulemaking (40 FR 47652) to revise the asbestos standard because the agency believed that "sufficient medical and scientific evidence has been accumulated to warrant the designation of asbestos as a human carcinogen," and that advances in monitoring and protective technology made reexamination of the standard "desirable." This proposal would have reduced the 8-h TWA to 0.5 f/cc, and imposed a ceiling limit of 5 f/cc for 15 min. The 1975 proposal would have applied to all industries except construction
7/76	OSHA's 8-h TWA limit was reduced to 2 f/cc
6/86	OSHA issued two revised standards, one governing occupational exposure to asbestos in general industry workplaces, the other applicable to construction workplaces
7/86	The revised standards amended OSHA's previous asbestos standard issued in 1972. The 1986 standards explicitly applied to occupational exposure to nonasbestiform tremolite, anthophyllite, and actinolite. After a subsequent and separate rulemaking proceeding, OSHA has deleted these minerals from the scope of the asbestos standards
?/86	The separate comprehensive asbestos standards for general industry and construction which were issued in 1986 shared the same permissible exposure limit (PEL) and most ancillary requirements. Both standards reduced the 8-h time weighted average (TWA) PEL 10-fold to 0.2 f/cc from the previous 2 f/cc limit. Specific provisions were added in the construction standard to cover unique hazards relating to asbestos abatement and demolition jobs
2/88	The US Court of Appeals for the District of Columbia issued its decision upholding most major challenged provisions, but remanding certain issues to OSHA for reconsideration (BCTD, AFL-CIO v. Brock, 838 F.2d 1258). The court determined that OSHA had not adequately explained why it was not adopting certain recommended provisions in light of evidence suggesting that those provisions would be feasible to implement, and would provide more than a de Minimis benefit for worker's health. The court also ordered OSHA to clarify the regulatory text for two provisions and found one provision, a ban of spraying asbestos-containing products, unsupported by the record. In addition, OSHA's failure to adopt a short-term exposure limit (STEL) was ordered to be reconsidered within 60 days of the court's mandate
9/88	OSHA issued a STEL of 1 f/cc measured over a 30-min sampling period

assessment narrative, because the "decision" making, or risk characterization, is constantly under review based on the available data and information that is available. Thus, a risk assessment is never "complete" if the state of the science is always changing and evolving. This is a good application of the concept of the risk assessment framework, as explained in the EPA chapter and for those familiar with the NAS *Red Book*. What is also important to note in the risk assessment and risk management decision process is that stakeholders, namely the AFL-CIO in this case, used the legal system to influence the risk assessment process with court cases and decisions. The interaction of science and law is an interesting one, somewhat unique to the United States compared to other countries with governing bodies.

4.3 ONGOING CHALLENGES WITH OSHA AND ACGIH REGULATORY LIMITS

While the adoption of the thousands of ACGIH OSHA exposure limits in the 1970s helped to protect worker and public health, there has been a lot of concern and criticism that these have not been updated. The review and revision process is time and resource intensive, often calling on experts to provide extra time on top what is their normal occupation or process for compensation. The reader can note that the similar challenges exist with the conducting and evaluation / acceptance of risk assessment as with the EPAs IRIS process, where public engagement, updates based on new science and methodologies, and the expectations of transparency in decision making and criteria are expected.

FURTHER READING

http://www.acgih.org/about-us/history.

https://www.osha.gov/pls/oshaweb/owadisp.show_document?p_table=PREAMBLES&p_id=775.

CHAPTER 5

Risk Assessment in the 21st Century: New Technologies and Techniques

René Viñas and Ted W. Simon

SECTION 5.1

Big Data: Benefits and Challenges

René Viñas[1] and Ted W. Simon[2]
[1]Grocery Manufacturers Association, Washington, DC, United States
[2]Ted Simon LLC, Winston, GA, United States

Animal-based studies have traditionally been used in toxicological testing, primarily stemming from the lack of viable testing alternatives. However, for several decades, there has been a movement to strategically create efficient alternatives to animal testing that will not only enhance animal welfare, but also decrease the monetary costs of experimental testing (Zhu et al., 2014a, 2014b; Bratcher and Reinhard, 2015; NRC, 2007; Szymanski et al., 2012). Current efforts by various U.S. agencies to bring these novel methodologies into the mainstream have been the focus of several research programs, such as ToxCast and "Tox21" (Toxicology Testing in the 21st Century) (NRC, 2007). Examples of these alternatives include high-throughput (HTP) cell-based "-omics" technologies, *in silico* (e.g., QSAR) methodologies, and 3D "organ-on-a-chip" cell models (Tralau et al., 2015; Jackson and Lu, 2016).

The collaborative effort of these programs has the aim of developing in vitro methodologies to evaluate and prioritize chemicals for future animal testing based on their potential toxicological concerns (Zhu et al., 2014a, 2014b; Tralau et al., 2012, NRC, 2007). As mentioned in the National Research Council's (NRC) vision for a new paradigm in toxicological testing, the goal is also to keep up with the

History of Risk Assessment in Toxicology. DOI: http://dx.doi.org/10.1016/B978-0-12-809532-4.00006-0

"backlog of untested chemicals in commerce" (Kavlock et al., 2012; NRC, 2007). The consequence of these initiatives has generated a large amount of data sets, far exceeding management capabilities (Merelli et al., 2014); hence the term "Big Data."

Several challenges exist that limit the widespread integration and acceptance of big data by risk assessors and regulators. The arguments of *relevance* and *validation* of the observed effects in an in vitro system to a more complex whole organism is a common theme among regulators who consider in vivo testing as the gold standard (Tralau et al., 2012). This high expectation comes from the general practice of conducting two-generation animal studies which are used to determine the systemic, developmental, reproductive, and carcinogenic effects from the long-term exposure to a single chemical (Rovida and Hartung, 2009; OECD, 2001). Further tests on a second animal species are sometimes recommended (Tralau et al., 2012). A suggested solution to this problem may be a strategic combination of in vitro assays, as well as the use of "real-life" target organ doses (Tralau et al., 2015). Other issues that remain include the reliability (quantitatively and qualitatively) of an assay's reproducibility between different laboratory systems and over time, too few reference substances available to meet current validation guidelines, transparency in the process for the generation of data, and greater availability of databases, as many databases (e.g., ToxCast) are not publically available (Judson et al., 2013; Hartung, 2016; Kavlock et al,. 2012; Tralau et al., 2015). Lastly, when dealing with big data sets, good quality control and assurance practices are essential when entering data into the database. Random errors have been noted, for example, in the original dose-response ToxCast data (Zhu et al., 2014a, 2014b). As stated in a publication by Thomas Hartung on "Making Big Sense from Big Data..." *trash in, trash out* (Hartung, 2016).

REFERENCES

Bratcher, N., Reinhard., G.R., 2015. Creative implementation of 3Rs principles within industry programs: beyond regulations and guidelines. J. Am. Assoc. Lab. Anim. Sci. 54 (2), 133–138.

Hartung, T., 2016. Making big sense from big data in toxicology by read-across. ALTEX 33 (2), 83–93.

Jackson, E.L., Lu, H., 2016. Three-dimensional models for studying development and disease: moving on from organisms to organs-on a chip and organoids. Integr.Biol 8, 672–683. Available from: http://dx.doi.org/10.1039/c6ib00039h.

Judson, R., Kavlock, R., Matthew, M., Reif, D., Houck, K., Knudsen, T., et al., 2013. Perspectives on validation of high-throughput assays supporting 21st century toxicity testing. ALTEX 30, 51–66.

Kavlock, R., Chandler, K., Houck, K., Hunter, S., Judson, R., Kleinstreuer, N., et al., 2012. Update on EPA's ToxCast program: providing high throughput decision support tools for chemical risk management. Chem. Res. Toxicol. 25, 1287–1302. Available from: http://dx.doi.org/10.1021/tx3000939.

Rovida, C., Hartung, T., 2009. Re-evaluation of animal numbers and costs for in vivo tests to accomplish REACH legislation requirements for chemicals—a report by the transatlantic think tank for toxicology (t4). ALTEX 26, 187–208. Available at: http://www.altex.ch/Current-issue.50.html?iid = 107&aid = 4.

Merelli, I., Pérez-Sánchez, H., Gesing, S., D'Agostino, D., 2014. Managing, analysing, and integrating big data in medical bioinformatics: open problems and future perspectives. BioMed Res. Int. 2014, 1–13. Available at: http://dx.doi.org/10.1155/2014/134023.

NRC (National Research Council), 2007. Toxicity Testing in the 21st Century: A Vision and a Strategy. The National Academies Press, Washington DC, doi: 10.17226/11970. Available at: http://www.nap.edu/catalog/11970/toxicity-testing-in-the-21st-century-a-vision-and-a.

OECD (Organization for Economic Co-operation and Development). 2011. OECD Guidelines for the Testing of Chemicals, Section 4. Text No. 433: Extended One-Generation Reproductive Toxicity Study. Available at: http://www.oecd-ilibrary.org/environment/test-no-443-extended-one-generation-reproductive-toxicity-study_9789264122550-en.

Szymanski, P., Magdalena, M., Mikiciuk-Olasik, E., 2012. Adaption of high-throughput screening in drug discovery—toxicological screening tests. Int. J. Mol. Sci. 13, 427–452. Available from: http://dx.doi.org/10.3390/ijms13010427.

Tralau, T., Riebeling, C., Pirow, R., Oelgeschläger, M., Seiler, A., Liebsch, M., Luch, A., 2012. Wind of change challenges toxicological regulators. Environ. Health Perspect. 120, 1489–1494. Available: http://dx.doi.org/10.1289/ehp.1104782.

Tralau, T., Oelgeschläger, M., Gürtler, R., Heinemeyer, G., Herzler, M., Höfer, T., et al., 2015. Regulatory toxicology in the twenty-first century: challenges, perspectives and possible solutions. Arch. Toxicol. 89, 823–850. Available from: http://dx.doi.org/10.1007/s00204-015-1510-0.

Zhu, H., Zhang, J., Kim, M.T., Boison, A., Sedykh, A., Moran, K., 2014a. Big data in chemical toxicity research: the use of high-throughput screening assays to identify potential toxicants. Chem. Res. Toxicol. 27, 1643–1651.

Zhu, H., Kim, M., Zhang, L., Sedykh, A., 2014b. Computers instead of cells: computational modeling of chemical toxicity. In: Allen, D., Waters, M.D. (Eds.), Reducing, Refining and Replacing the Use of Animals in Toxicity Testing. The Royal Society of Chemistry, Cambridge, pp. 163–182. (Chapter 5).

SECTION 5.2

Evidence-Based Toxicology Versus Weight of Evidence in Influencing Risk Assessment: Design and Approach

René Viñas[1] and Ted W. Simon[2]
[1]Grocery Manufacturers Association, Washington, DC, United States
[2]Ted Simon LLC, Winston, GA, United States

A weight of evidence (WOE) approach is used by authoritative bodies (e.g., EPA, FDA) to assess the strength of the scientific reasoning that can be taken from a given body of evidence (NRC, 2009). Typically, WOE is used in circumstances where there is an appreciable level of uncertainty, and is used to determine whether the supporting evidence for one side of the case, or argument, is greater over the supporting evidence for the other, after an unbiased assessment. The EPA, for example, relies on peer reviews from groups of experts to use WOE when evaluating the hazards of a given chemical (toxic or carcinogenic), and is used to describe the strength of the evidence that supports modes of action and dose−response relationships (NRC, 2009).

The use of WOE can be controversial, as there is no standard procedure to follow, nor is there a clear definition of the term. Much of the criticism surrounding WOE approaches include the issue of being non-transparent, having inconsistent decision-making procedures for hazard and risk assessments for individual chemicals, and having a reliance on aged toxicological methods with an unclear performance (Stephens et al., 2013). Without a clear method in place, the process could lead to a highly subjective process (Hartung, 2009). In a 2005 article, Douglas L. Weed conducted an extensive review characterizing the use of the phrase "weight of evidence" (Weed, 2005). After reviewing 276 papers for the years 1994 through 2004, Weed identified several problems which involved the multiple use and lack of consensus for the term "weight of evidence," as well as a constant lack of a definition for the term itself and the various kinds of weights, both qualitative and quantitative, which can be used in risk assessment (Weed, 2005).

In order to ensure unbiased review procedures, institutions such as the EPA, the National Toxicology Program (NTP), the International Agency for Research on Cancer (IARC), and others, have developed procedures and classification systems to aid in reaching conclusions and consensus about the overall evidence, including convening expert bodies to perform WOE analyses (NRC, 2009). Much confusion about the process still exists, despite implementations to set controls (Hartung, 2009; Weed, 2005).

Stemming from Evidence-Based Medicine (EBM), Evidence-Based Toxicology (EBT) has a different approach to the traditional narrative review of WOE which tends to be biased and may rely on professional judgment (Hartung, 2009; Guzelain et al., 2005; Teagarden, 1989). The primary components of evidence-based methodologies are systematic reviews (Balls et al., 2006; Guzelain et al., 2005). Systematic reviews are a different type of literature review, in the sense that they appraise and synthesize the evidence in a systematic way, according to a predefined methodology to maximize the precision of conclusions, while avoiding bias (Guzelain et al., 2005). The methodologies with which systematic reviews are carried out differ from a narrative review in a variety of ways: (1) framing of the question to be addressed is narrower in focus; (2) there is a criteria to identifying relevant studies and also which studies will be excluded from the analysis; (3) how the chosen studies will be appraised for their risk of bias/quality, and how the data will be combined and synthesized across the multiple studies (i.e., meta-analysis). A protocol is usually developed prior to initiating data collection (Horvath and Pewsner, 2004).

Critical appraisal of the data in a manner that is transparent, unbiased, and consistent, is the goal of an evidence-based approach (Stephens et al., 2013). Actions to promote and familiarize personnel with the use of EBT are currently under way. One such action is the establishment of the Evidence-Based Toxicology Collaboration (EBTC). Founded in 2011 at Johns Hopkins University, EBTC brings together interested stakeholders to work on methodological challenges and apply evidence-based approaches to public health problems (www.ebtox.org).

REFERENCES

Balls, M., Amcoff, P., Bremer, S., Casati, S., Coecke, S., Clothier, R., et al., 2006. The principles of weigh of evidence validation of test methods and testing strategies: the report and recommendations of ECVAM workshop 58a. Altern. Lab. Anim. 34 (6), 603–620.

Guzelain, P.S., Victoroff, M.S., Halmes, N.C., James, R.C., Guzelian, C.P., 2005. Evidence-based toxicology: a comprehensive framework for causation. Hum. Exp. Toxicol. 24, 161–201.

Hartung, T., 2009. Food for thought...on evidence-based toxicology. ALTEX 26, 75–82.

Horvath, A.R., Pewsner, D., 2004. Systematic reviews in laboratory medicine: principles, processes and practical considerations. Clin. Chim. Acta 342, 23–39.

NRC (National Research Council), 2009. Science and Decisions: Advancing Risk Assessment. The National Academies Press, Washington DC, ISBN: 0-309-12047-0, Available: http://www.nap.edu/catalog/12209.html.

Stephens, M.L., Andersen, M., Becker, R.A., Kellyn, B., Boekelheide, K., Carney, E., et al., 2013. Evidence-based toxicology for the 21st century: opportunities and challenges. ALTEX 30, 74–103.

Teagarden, J.R., 1989. Meta-analysis: Whither narrative review? Pharmacotherapy 9, 274–284.

Weed, D.L., 2005. Weight of evidence: a review of concept and methods. Risk Anal. 25, 1545–1557.

Printed in the United States
By Bookmasters

Printed in the United States
By Bookmasters